The Joy of Plants

Step by Step Simple Plant-Based Recipes for
a Happy Mind and a Healthy Body

The Green Solution

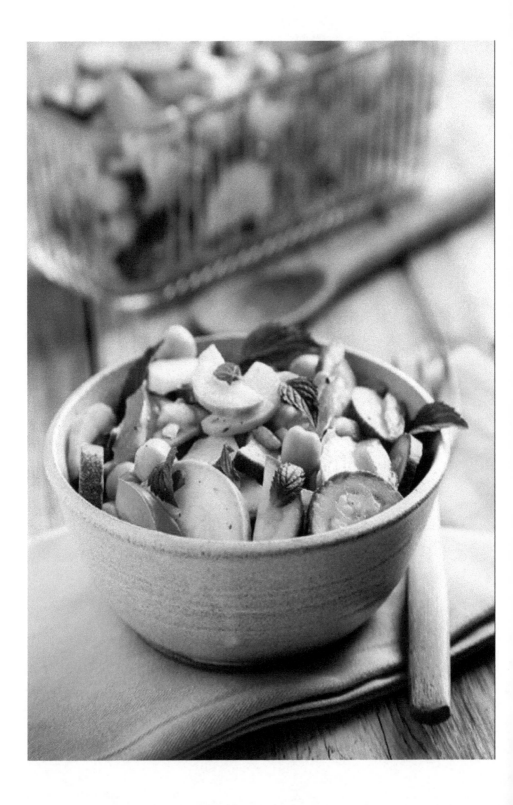

Table of Contents

INTRODUCTION

A plant-based diet is a diet consisting mostly or entirely of plant-based foods with no animal products or artificial ingredients. While a plant-based diet avoids or has limited animal products, it is not necessarily vegan. This includes not only fruits and vegetables, but also nuts, seeds, oils, whole grains, legumes, and beans. It doesn't mean that you are vegetarian or vegan and never eat meat, eggs, or dairy.

Vegetarian diets have also been shown to support health, including a lower risk of developing coronary heart disease, high blood pressure, diabetes, and increased longevity.

Plant-based diets offer all the necessary carbohydrates, vitamins, protein, fats, and minerals for optimal health, and are often higher in fiber and phytonutrients. However, some vegans may need to add a supplement to ensure they receive all the nutrients required.

Who says that plant-based diets are limited or boring? There are lots of delicious recipes that you can use to make mouthwatering, healthy, plant-based dishes that will satisfy your cravings. If you're eating these plant-based foods regularly, you can maintain a healthy weight without obsessing about calories and avoid diseases that result from bad dietary habits.

Benefits of a Plant-Based Diet

Eating a plant-based diet improves the health of your gut so you are better able to absorb the nutrients from food that support your immune system and reduce inflammation. Fiber can lower cholesterol and stabilize blood sugar, and it's great for good bowel management.

- **A Plant-Based Diet May Lower Your Blood Pressure**
  High blood pressure, or hypertension, can increase the risk for health issues, including heart disease, stroke, and type 2 diabetes and reduce blood pressure and other risky conditions.

- **A Plant-Based Diet May Keep Your Heart Healthy**
  Saturated fat in meat can contribute to heart issues when eaten in excess, so plant-based foods can help keep your heart healthy.

- **A Plant-Based Diet May Help Prevent Type 2 Diabetes**
  Animal foods can increase cholesterol levels, so eating a plant-based diet filled with high-quality plant foods can reduce the risk of developing type 2 diabetes by 34 percent.

- **Eating a Plant-Based Diet Could Help You Lose Weight**
  Cutting back on meat can help you to maintain a healthy weight because a plant-based diet is naturally satisfying and rich in fiber.

- **Following a Plant-Based Diet Long Term May Help You Live Longer**
  If you stick with healthy plant-based foods your whole body will be leaner and healthier, allowing you to stay healthy and vital as you age.

- **A Plant-Based Diet May Decrease Your Risk of Cancer**
  Vegetarians have an 18 percent lower risk of cancer compared to non-vegetarians. This is because a plant-based diet is rich of fibers and healthy nutrients.

- **A Plant-Based Diet May Improve Your Cholesterol**
  High cholesterol can lead to fatty deposits in the blood, which can restrict blood flow and potentially lead to heart attack, stroke, heart disease, and many other problems. A plant-based diet can help in maintaining healthy cholesterol levels.

- **Ramping Up Your Plant Intake May Keep Your Brain Strong**
  Increased consumption of fruits and vegetables is associated with a 20 percent reduction in the risk of cognitive impairment and dementia. So plant foods can help protect your brain from multiple issues.

What to Eat in Plant-Based Diets

Fruits: Berries, citrus fruits, pears, peaches, pineapple, bananas, etc.

Vegetables: Kale, spinach, tomatoes, broccoli, cauliflower, carrots, asparagus, peppers, etc.

Starchy vegetables: Potatoes, sweet potatoes, butternut squash, etc.

Whole grains: Brown rice, rolled oats, farro, quinoa, brown rice pasta, barley, etc.

Healthy fats: Avocados, olive oil, coconut oil, unsweetened coconut, etc.

Legumes: Peas, chickpeas, lentils, peanuts, black beans, etc.

Seeds, nuts, and nut butters: Almonds, cashews, macadamia nuts, pumpkin seeds, sunflower seeds, natural peanut butter, tahini, etc.

Unsweetened plant-based milks: Coconut milk, almond milk, cashew milk, etc.

Spices, herbs, and seasonings: Basil, rosemary, turmeric, curry, black pepper, salt, etc.

Condiments: Salsa, mustard, nutritional yeast, soy sauce, vinegar, lemon juice, etc.

Plant-based protein: Tofu, tempeh, plant-based protein sources or powders with no added sugar or artificial ingredients.

Beverages: Coffee, tea, sparkling water, etc.

What Not to Eat in Plant-Based Diets

Fast food: French fries, cheeseburgers, hot dogs, chicken nuggets, etc.

Added sugars and sweets: Table sugar, soda, juice, pastries, cookies, candy, sweet tea, sugary cereals, etc.

Refined grains: White rice, white pasta, white bread, bagels, etc.

Packaged and convenience foods: Chips, crackers, cereal bars, frozen dinners, etc.

Processed vegan-friendly foods: Plant-based meats like; Tofurkey, faux cheeses, vegan butters, etc.

Artificial sweeteners: Equal, Splenda, Sweet'N Low, etc.

Processed animal products: Bacon, lunch meats, sausage, beef jerky, etc.

Day 1:

Breakfast (304 calories)

- 1 serving Berry-Kefir Smoothie

A.M. Snack (95 calories)

- 1 medium apple

Lunch (374 calories)

- 1 serving Green Salad with Pita Bread & Hummus

P.M. Snack (206 calories)

- 1/4 cup dry-roasted unsalted almonds

Dinner (509 calories)

- 1 serving Beefless Vegan Tacos
- 2 cups mixed greens
- 1 serving Citrus Vinaigrette

Day 2:

Breakfast (258 calories)

- 1 serving Cinnamon Roll Overnight Oats
- 1 medium orange

A.M. Snack (341 calories)

- 1 cup low-fat plain Greek yogurt
- 1 medium peach
- 3 Tbsps slivered almonds

Lunch (332 calories)

- 1 serving Thai-Style Chopped Salad with Sriracha Tofu

P.M. Snack (131 calories)

- 1 large pear

Dinner (458 calories)

- 1 serving Mexican Quinoa Salad

Day 3:

Breakfast (258 calories)

- 1 serving Cinnamon Roll Overnight Oats
- 1 medium orange

A.M. Snack (95 calories)

- 1 medium apple

Lunch (463 calories)

- 1 serving Thai-Style Chopped Salad with Sriracha Tofu
- 1 large pear

P.M. Snack (274 calories)

- 1/3 cup dried walnut halves
- 1 medium peach

Dinner (419 calories)

- 1 serving Eggs in Tomato Sauce with Chickpeas & Spinach
- 1 1-oz. slice whole-wheat baguette

BREAKFAST

Raspberry Raisins Muffins with Orange Glaze

Servings: 8

Preparation Time: 55 minutes

Per Serving: Calories 700 Fats 25.5g Carbs 115.1g Protein 10. 5g

Ingredients:

For the muffins:

- 4 tsps vanilla extract
- 4 cups whole-wheat flour
- 3 tsps baking powder
- 4 tbsps flax seed powder + 12 tbsps water
- 1 cup plant butter, room temperature
- 2 cups pure date sugar
- 1 cup oat milk
- 2 pinches of salt
- 2 lemons, zested
- 2 cups dried raspberries

For the orange glaze:

- 4 tbsps orange juice
- 2 cups pure date sugar

Procedure:

1. First, preheat the oven to 400 F and grease 6 muffin cups with cooking spray.
2. Take a small bowl, mix the flax seed powder with water and allow thickening for 5 minutes to make the flax egg.
3. Take a medium bowl; mix the flour, baking powder, and salt.
4. Take another bowl, cream the plant butter, date sugar, and flax egg. Mix in the oat milk, vanilla, and lemon zest.
5. Then, combine both mixtures, fold in raspberries, and fill muffin cups two-thirds way up with the batter.
6. Now, bake until a toothpick inserted comes out clean, 20-25 minutes.
7. Take a medium bowl, whisk orange juice, and date sugar until smooth. Remove the muffins when ready and transfer them to a wire rack to cool.
8. Drizzle the glaze on top to serve.

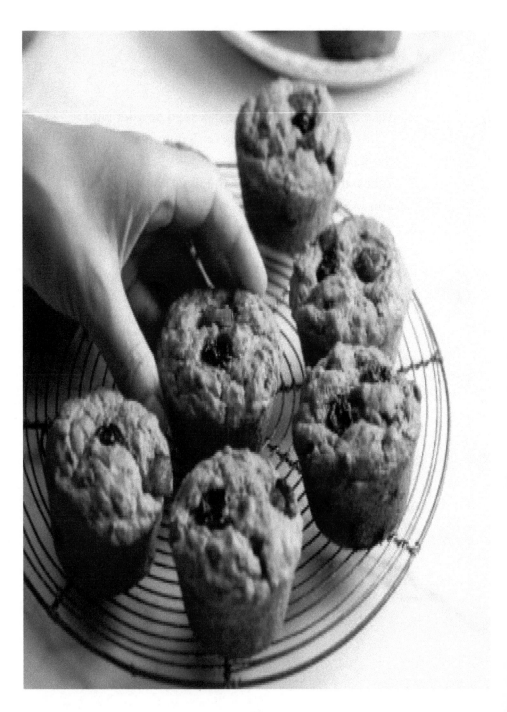

Breakfast Vegan Breakfast Muffins

Servings: 4

Preparation Time: 30 minutes

Per Serving: Carbs: 18g Protein: 12g Fats: 14g Calories: 276 Kcal

Ingredients:

- 1 Avocado peeled and sliced
- 2 Sliced fresh tomatoes
- 5-6 tablespoons Romesco Sauce
- 4 tofu scramble
- 1 cup fresh baby spinach
- 4 Vegan English muffins

Procedure:

1. In the oven, toast the English muffin
2. Then, half the muffin and spread romesco sauce
3. Paste spinach to one side, tailed by avocado slices
4. Now, have warm tofu followed by a tomato slice
5. Finally, place the other muffin half onto to the preceding one

Easy Almond Waffles with Cranberries

Servings: 8

Preparation Time: 40 minutes

Per Serving: Calories 533 Fats 53g Carbs 16. 7g Protein 1.2g

Ingredients:

- 4 tbsps flax seed powder + 12 tbsps water
- 1/4 cup almond flour
- 2 cups fresh almond butter
- 4 tbsps pure maple syrup
- 2 tsps fresh lemon juice
- 5 tsps baking powder
- 2 pinches salt
- 3 cups almond milk
- 4 tbsps plant butter

Procedure:

1. Take a medium bowl, mix the flax seed powder with water and allow soaking for 5 minutes.
2. Then, add the almond flour, baking powder, salt, and almond milk. Mix until well combined.
3. Preheat a waffle iron and brush with some plant butter.
4. Pour in a quarter cup of the batter, close the iron and cook until the waffles are golden and crisp, 2 to 3 minutes.

5. Transfer the waffles to a plate and make more waffles using the same process and ingredient proportions.
6. Meanwhile, in a medium bowl, mix the almond butter with maple syrup and lemon juice.
7. Finally, serve the waffles, spread the top with the almond-lemon mixture, and serve.

Chickpea Omelet with Spinach & Mushrooms

Servings: 8

Preparation Time: 35 minutes

Per Serving: Calories 147 Fats 1. 8g Carbs 21.3g Protein 11.6g

Ingredients:

- 6 scallions, chopped
- 2 cups sautéed sliced white button mushrooms
- 1 cup chopped fresh spinach
- 2 cups halved cherry tomatoes for serving
- 2 cups chickpea flour
- 1 tsp onion powder
- 1 tsp garlic powder
- 1/2 tsp white pepper
- 1/2 tsp black pepper
- 1/4 cup nutritional yeast
- 1 tsp baking soda
- 2 small green bell peppers, deseeded and chopped
- 2 tbsps fresh parsley leaves

Procedure:

1. Take a medium bowl, mix the chickpea flour, onion powder, garlic powder, white pepper, black

pepper, nutritional yeast, and baking soda until well combined.

2. Then, heat a medium skillet over medium heat and add a quarter of the batter.

3. Swirl the pan to spread the batter across the pan.

4. After that, scatter a quarter each of the bell pepper, scallions, mushrooms, and spinach on top, and cook until the bottom part of the omelet sets and is golden brown, 1 to 2 minutes.

5. Now, carefully, flip the omelet and cook the other side until set and golden brown.

6. Transfer the omelet to a plate and make the remaining omelets using the remaining batter in the same proportions.

7. Finally, serve the omelet with the tomatoes and garnish with the parsley leaves. Serve.

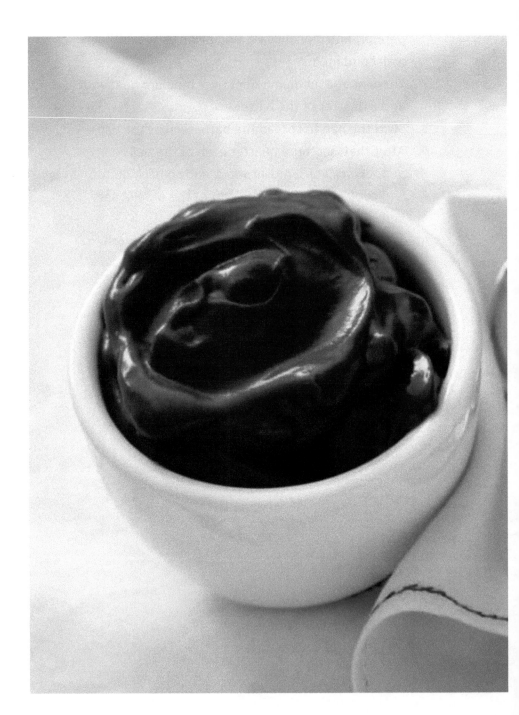

Morning Raw Pudding

Servings: 6

Preparation Time: 10 minutes

Per Serving: Calories: 364; Fat: 10.5g; Carbs: 61.4g; Protein: 9g

Ingredients:

- 5 cups almond milk
- 2 pinches of grated nutmeg
- 1/2 teaspoons ground cardamom
- 1/2 teaspoons crystalized ginger
- 6 tablespoons agave syrup
- 1 teaspoon vanilla essence
- 2 pinches of flaky salt
- 1 cup instant oats
- 1 cup chia seeds

Procedure:

1. First, add the milk, agave syrup, and spices to a bowl and stir until everything is well incorporated.
2. Then, fold in the instant oats and chia seeds and stir again to combine well.
3. Now, spoon the mixture into three jars, cover, and place it in your refrigerator overnight.
4. On the actual day, stir with a spoon and serve.

Healthy Lemony Quinoa Muffins

Servings: 10

Preparation Time: 25 minutes

Ingredients:

- 4 cups unsweetened lemon curd
- 1 cup pure date sugar
- 4 tbsps coconut oil melted, plus more for coating the muffin tin
- ½ cup ground flaxseed
- 5 cups whole-wheat flour
- 3 cups cooked quinoa
- 4 tsps baking soda
- 2 pinches of salt
- 2 tsps apple cider vinegar
- 1 cup raisins

Procedure:

1. First of all, preheat the oven to 400 F.
2. Then, take a bowl, combine the flaxseed and ½ cup water.
3. Stir in the lemon curd, sugar, coconut oil, and vinegar.
4. Now, add in flour, quinoa, baking soda, and salt. Put in the raisins, be careful not too fluffy.
5. Divide the batter between greased with coconut oil cups of the tin and bake for 20 minutes until golden and set. Allow cooling slightly before removing it from the tin. Serve.

Pecan & Pear Farro

Servings: 8

Preparation Time: 20 minutes

Ingredients:

- 2 cups farro
- 4 cups water
- 4 pears, peeled, cored, and chopped
- 1/2 cup chopped pecans
- 1 tsp salt
- 2 tbsps plant butter

Procedure:

1. First, bring water to a boil in a pot over high heat.
2. Stir in salt and farro.
3. Lower the heat, cover, and simmer for 15 minutes until the farro is tender and the liquid has absorbed.
4. Then, turn the heat off and add in the butter, pears, and pecans.
5. Cover and rest for 12-15 minutes. Serve immediately.

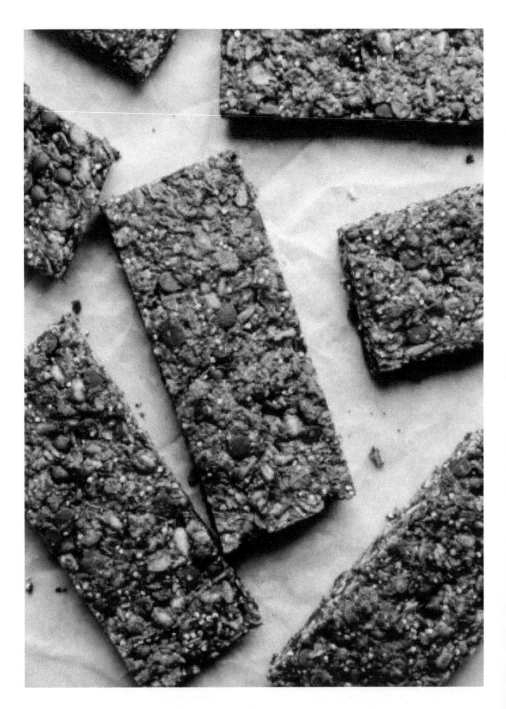

Morning Chocolate Granola Bars

Servings: 24

Preparation Time: 40 minutes

Per Serving: Calories: 229; Fat: 13.4g; Carbs: 27.9g; Protein: 3.1g

Ingredients:

- 1 cup almonds
- 1 cup walnuts
- 1/2 cup almond butter, room temperature
- 4 tablespoons coconut oil, melted
- 2 pinches of grated nutmeg
- 1 cup dark chocolate chunks
- 1/2 cup pecans
- 1 teaspoon allspice
- 2 pinches of salt
- 2 1/2 cups old-fashioned oats
- 1 cup fresh dates, pitted and mashed
- 1 cup dried cherries
- 1/2 cup agave syrup

Procedure:

1. Take a mixing bowl, thoroughly combine the oats, dates, and dried cherries.
2. Then, add in the agave syrup, almond butter, and coconut oil. Stir in the nuts, spices, and chocolate.

3. Now, press the mixture into a lightly greased baking dish.
4. Transfer it to your refrigerator for about 30 minutes.
5. Slice into 12 even bars and store in airtight containers.

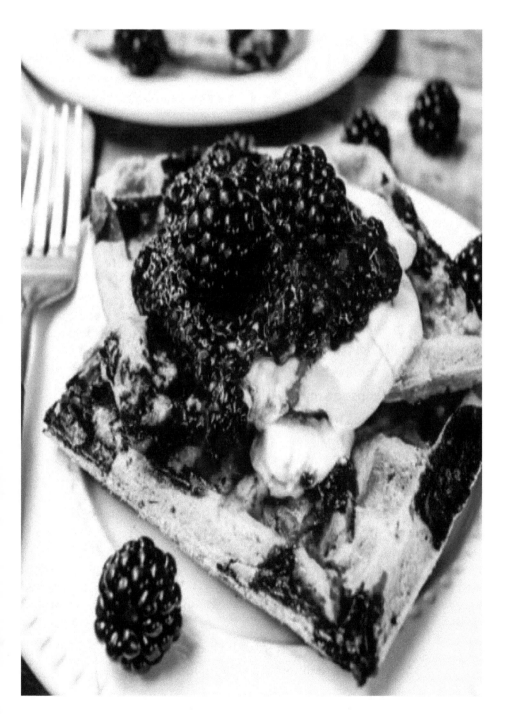

Easy Blackberry Waffle

Servings: 8

Preparation Time: 15 minutes

Ingredients:

- 1 cup old-fashioned oats
- 1/2 cup date sugar
- 6 tsps baking powder
- 1 tsp salt
- 2 tsps ground cinnamon
- 3 cups whole-wheat flour
- 2 tsps lemon zest
- 1/2 cup plant butter, melted
- 1 cup fresh blackberries
- 4 cups soy milk
- 2 tbsps fresh lemon juice

Procedure:

1. First, preheat the waffle iron.
2. Take a bowl, mix flour, oats, sugar, baking powder, salt, and cinnamon. Set aside.
3. Take another bowl, combine milk, lemon juice, lemon zest, and butter.
4. Pour into the wet ingredients and whisk to combine.
5. Now, add the butter to the hot greased waffle iron, using approximately a ladleful for each waffle.

6. Then, cook for 3-5 minutes, until golden brown.
7. Repeat the process until no batter is left.
8. Finally, serve topped with blackberries

Apple & Almond Buckwheat Porridge

Servings: 6

Preparation Time: 20 minutes

Per Serving: Calories: 377; Fat: 8.8g; Carbs: 70g; Protein: 10.6g

Ingredients:

- 2 cups rice milk
- 1/2 teaspoons sea salt
- 6 tablespoons agave syrup
- 2 cups apples, cored and diced
- 6 tablespoons almonds, slivered
- 2 cups buckwheat groats, toasted
- 1 1/2 cups water
- 4 tablespoons coconut flakes
- 4 tablespoons hemp seeds

Procedure:

1. Take a saucepan, bring the buckwheat groats, water, milk, and salt to a boil.
2. Then, immediately turn the heat to a simmer; let it simmer for about 13 minutes until it has softened.
3. Now, stir in the agave syrup. Divide the porridge between three serving bowls.
4. Then, garnish each serving with apples, almonds, coconut, and hemp seeds.

Spanish Tortilla

Servings: 4

Preparation Time: 35 minutes

Per Serving: Calories: 379; Fat: 20.6g; Carbs: 45.2g;
Protein: 5.6g

Ingredients:

- 4 medium potatoes, peeled and diced
- 16 tablespoons water
- Sea salt and ground black pepper, to season
- 1 teaspoon Spanish paprika
- 6 tablespoons olive oil
- 1 white onion, chopped
- 16 tablespoons gram flour

Procedure:

1. First of all, heat 4 tablespoons of olive oil in a frying pan over a moderate flame.
2. Now, cook the potatoes and onion; cook for about 20 minutes or until tender; reserve.
3. Then, take a mixing bowl, thoroughly combine the flour, water, salt, black pepper, and paprika.
4. Then, add in the potato/onion mixture.
5. Heat the remaining 2 tablespoons of olive oil in the same frying pan.

6. Pour 1/2 of the batter into the frying pan.
7. Cook your tortilla for about 11 minutes, turning it once or twice to promote even cooking.
8. Then, repeat with the remaining batter and serve warm.

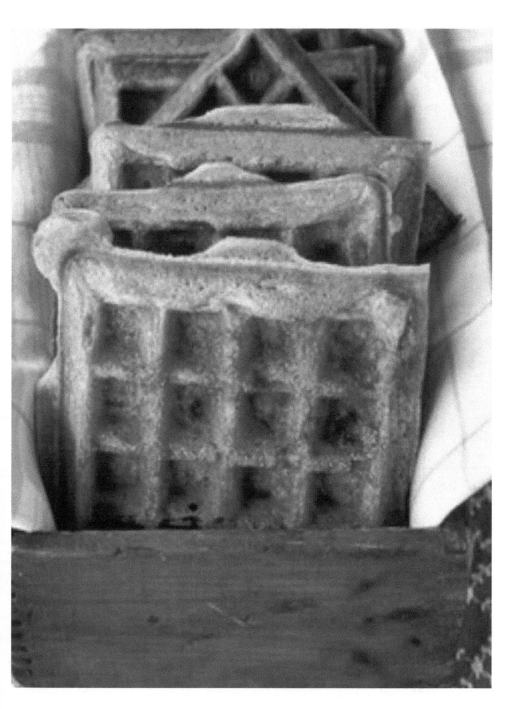

Morning Gingerbread Belgian Waffles

Servings: 6

Preparation Time: 25 minutes

Per Serving: Calories: 299; Fat: 12.6g; Carbs: 38.5g; Protein: 6.8g

Ingredients:

- 2 teaspoons ground ginger
- 2 cups almond milk
- 4 tbsps olive oil
- 2 teaspoons vanilla extract
- 2 cups all-purpose flour
- 2 teaspoons baking powder
- 2 tablespoons brown sugar

Procedure:

1. First, preheat a waffle iron according to the manufacturer's instructions.
2. Take a mixing bowl, thoroughly combine the flour, baking powder, brown sugar, ground ginger, almond milk, vanilla extract, and olive oil.
3. Then, beat until everything is well blended.
4. Now, ladle 1/3 of the batter into the preheated waffle iron and cook until the waffles are golden and crisp.
5. Repeat with the remaining batter.
6. Serve your waffles with blackberry jam, if desired.

Banana& Walnut Porridge

Servings: 8

Preparation Time: 15 minutes

Per Serving: Calories: 389; Fat: 11.6g; Carbs: 67.7g; Protein: 16.8g

Ingredients:

- 4 cups unsweetened almond milk
- 8 tablespoons agave nectar
- 2 cups rolled oats
- 2 cups spelt flakes
- 8 tablespoons walnuts, chopped
- 4 bananas, sliced

Procedure:

1. Take a nonstick skillet, fry the oats, and spelt flakes until fragrant, working in batches.
2. Then, bring the milk to a boil and add in the oats, spelt flakes, and agave nectar.
3. Turn the heat to a simmer and let it cook for 6 to 7 minutes, stirring occasionally.
4. Now, top with walnuts and bananas and serve warm.

SALADS

Homemade Baked Sweet Potatoes With Corn Salad

Servings: 8

Preparation Time: 15-30 minutes

Per Serving: Calories 372 Fats 20. 7g Carbs 41. 7g Protein 8. 9g

Ingredients:

For the baked sweet potatoes:

- 4 scallions, thinly sliced
- 4 limes, juiced
- 6 tbsps olive oil
- Salt and black pepper to taste
- 8 medium sweet potatoes, peeled and cut into ½-inch cubes
- 1/2 tsp cayenne pepper

For the corn salad:

- 2 (3 oz.) cans of sweet corn kernels, drained
- 2 tsps cumin powder
- 1 tbsp plant butter, melted
- 2 large green chilies, deseeded and minced

Procedure:

For the baked sweet potatoes:

1. First, preheat the oven to 400 F and lightly grease a baking sheet with cooking spray.
2. Take a medium bowl, add the sweet potatoes, lime juice, salt, black pepper, and cayenne pepper.
3. Now, toss well and spread the mixture on the baking sheet.
4. Then, bake in the oven until the potatoes soften, 20 to 25 minutes.
5. Finally, remove from the oven, transfer to a serving plate, and garnish with the scallions.

For the corn salad:

1. Take a medium bowl, mix the corn kernels, butter, green chili, and cumin powder.
2. Now, serve the sweet potatoes with the corn salad.

Healthy Cashew Siam Salad

Servings: 8

Preparation Time: 10 minutes

Per Serving: Calories 236 Carbohydrates 6. 1 g Fats 21. 6 g Protein 4. 2 g

Ingredients:

Salad:

- 1 cup pickled red cabbage
- 8 cups baby spinach, rinsed, drained

Dressing:

- 6 tbsps avocado oil
- 2 tbsps soy sauce
- 2-inch piece ginger, finely chopped
- 2 tsps chili garlic paste
- 1 tbsp rice vinegar
- 1 tbsp sesame oil

Toppings:

- 1/2 cup fresh cilantro, chopped
- 1 cup raw cashews, unsalted

Procedure:

1. First, put the spinach and red cabbage in a large bowl.

2. Now, toss to combine and set the salad aside.
3. Then, toast the cashews in a frying pan over medium-high heat, occasionally stirring until the cashews are golden brown. This should take about 3 minutes.
4. After that, turn off the heat and set the frying pan aside.
5. Now, mix all the dressing ingredients in a medium-sized bowl and use a spoon to mix them into a smooth dressing.
6. Then, pour the dressing over the spinach salad and top with the toasted cashews.
7. Toss the salad to combine all ingredients and transfer the large bowl to the fridge.
8. Allow the salad to chill for up to one hour – doing so will guarantee a better flavor.
9. Alternatively, the salad can be served right away, topped with the optional cilantro. Enjoy!

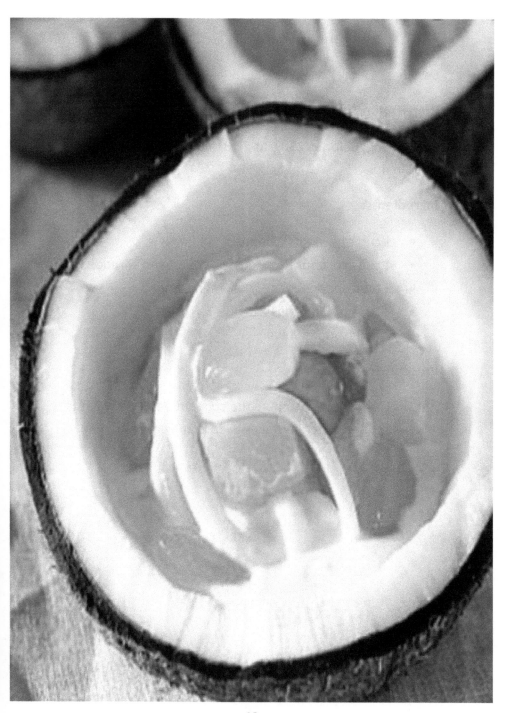

Delicious Coconut Salad

Servings: 12

Preparation Time: 10 minutes

Per Serving: Calories 250, Fat 23.8, Fiber 5.8, Carbs 8.9, Protein 4.5

Ingredients:

- 1 cup of walnuts, chopped
- 4 cups coconut flesh, unsweetened and shredded
- 2 tablespoons coconut oil, melted
- 2 cups blackberries
- 2 tablespoons stevia

Procedure:

1. Take a bowl, combine the coconut with the walnuts and the other ingredients, toss and serve.

Amazing Spinach and Mashed Tofu Salad

Servings: 8

Preparation Time: 20 minutes

Per Serving: Calories 166 Carbohydrates 5. 5 g Fats 10. 7 g Protein 11. 3 g

Ingredients:

- 3 tbsps soy sauce
- 4 tbsps water
- 8 cups baby spinach leaves
- 8 tbsps cashew butter
- 2 tsps nori flakes
- 2-inch piece ginger, finely chopped
- 56-oz. blocks firm tofu, drained
- 2 tsps red miso paste
- 4 tbsps sesame seeds
- 2 tsps organic orange zest

Procedure:

2. First, use paper towels to absorb any excess water left in the tofu before crumbling both blocks into small pieces.
3. Take a large bowl, combine the mashed tofu with the spinach leaves.
4. Now, mix the remaining ingredients in another small bowl and, if desired, add the optional water for a more smooth dressing.

5. Then, pour this dressing over the mashed tofu and spinach leaves.
6. Now, transfer the bowl to the fridge and allow the salad to chill for up to one hour.
7. Doing so will guarantee a better flavor. Or, the salad can be served right away. Enjoy!

Tasty Cucumber Edamame Salad

Servings: 4

Preparation Time: 5 minutes

Per Serving: Calories 409 Carbohydrates 7. 1 g Fats 38. 25 g Protein 7. 6 g

Ingredients:

- 6 tbsps avocado oil
- 2 cups cucumber, sliced into thin rounds
- 1 cup fresh sugar snap peas, sliced or whole
- 1 cup fresh edamame
- 1/2 cup radish, sliced
- 2 large Hass avocadoes, peeled, pitted, sliced
- 2 nori sheets, crumbled
- 4 tsps roasted sesame seeds
- 2 tsps salt

Procedure:

1. Bring a medium-sized pot filled halfway with water to a boil over medium-high heat.
2. Then, add the sugar snaps and cook them for about 2 minutes.
3. Now, take the pot off the heat, drain the excess water, transfer the sugar snaps to a medium-sized bowl, and set them aside for now.

4. Then, fill the pot with water again, add the teaspoon of salt and bring to a boil over medium-high heat.
5. Now, add the edamame to the pot and let them cook for about 6 minutes.
6. After, that takes the pot off the heat, drain the excess water, transfer the soybeans to the bowl with sugar snaps, and let them cool down for about 5 minutes.
7. Then, combine all ingredients, except the nori crumbs and roasted sesame seeds, in a medium-sized bowl.
8. Carefully stir, using a spoon, until all ingredients are evenly coated in oil.
9. Now, top the salad with the nori crumbs and roasted sesame seeds.
10. Then, transfer the bowl to the fridge and allow the salad to cool for at least 30 minutes.
11. In the end, serve chilled and enjoy!

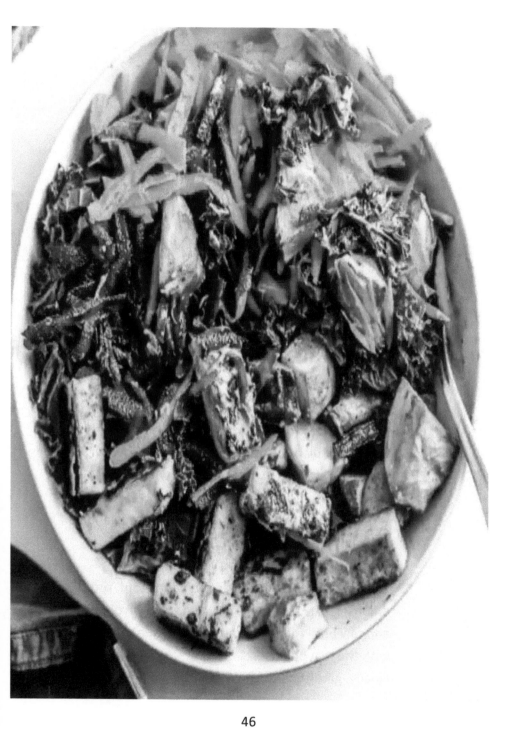

Amazing Beet Tofu Salad

Servings: 8

Preparation Time: 50 minutes

Ingredients:

- 4 oz. tofu, chopped into little bits
- 4 tbsps plant butter
- 16 oz. red beets
- 2 small romaine lettuce, torn
- Freshly chopped chives
- Salt and black pepper to taste
- 1 red onion
- 2 cups tofu mayonnaise

Procedure:

1. First, put beets in a pot, cover with water, and bring to a boil for 40 minutes.
2. Now, melt plant butter in a nonstick pan over medium heat and fry tofu until browned.
3. Then, set aside to cool.
4. When the bits are ready, drain through a colander and allow cooling.
5. Slip the skin off after, and slice them.
6. Take a salad bowl, combine the beets, tofu, red onions, lettuce, salt, pepper, and tofu mayonnaise and mix until the vegetables are adequately coated with the mayonnaise.
7. Finally, garnish with chives and serve.

Amazing Savory Pasta Salad with Cannellini Beans

Servings: 8

Preparation Time: 35 minutes

Ingredients:

- 2 medium zucchinis, sliced
- 4 garlic cloves, minced
- 5 cups whole-wheat bow tie pasta
- 1 cup crumbled tofu cheese
- 2 tbsps olive oil
- 4 large tomatoes, chopped
- 2 (30 oz.) cans cannellini beans
- 2 (4,1/2 oz.) can green olives, sliced

Procedure:

1. First, cook the pasta until al dente, 10 minutes.
2. Drain and set aside.
3. Now, heat olive oil in a skillet and sauté zucchini and garlic for 4 minutes.
4. Then, stir in tomatoes, beans, and olives.
5. Cook until the tomatoes soften, 10 minutes.
6. Mix in pasta.
7. After, that allows warming for 1 minute.
8. In the end, stir in tofu cheese and serve warm.

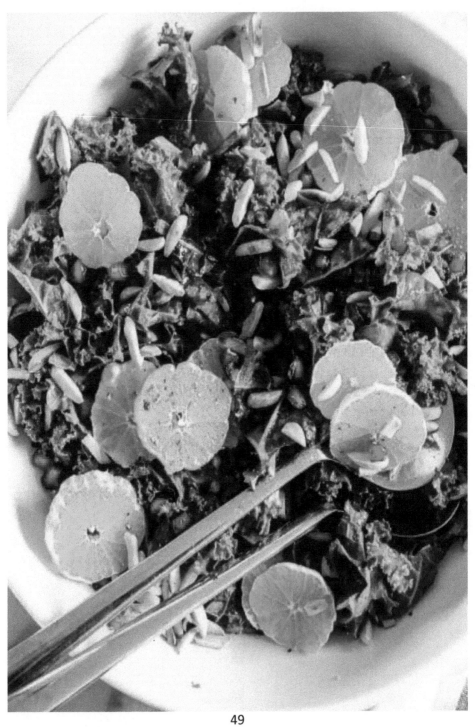

Healthy Orange & Kale Salad

Servings: 8

Preparation Time: 10 minutes

Ingredients:

- 4 tbsps olive oil
- 4 tbsps Dijon mustard
- 1/2 cup fresh orange juice
- 2 tsps agave nectar
- 2 oranges, peeled and segmented
- 1 red onion, sliced paper-thin
- 4 tbsps minced fresh parsley
- 2 tbsps minced green onions
- 8 cups fresh kale, chopped

Procedure:

1. Take a food processor; place the mustard, oil, orange juice, agave nectar, salt, pepper, parsley, and green onions.
2. Now, blend until smooth.
3. Set aside.
4. Take a bowl, combine the kale, orange, and onion.
5. Then, pour over the dressing and toss to coat.
6. Finally, serve.

Homemade African zucchini Salad

Servings: 4

Preparation Time: 20 minutes

Ingredients:

- 2 lemons, half zested and juiced, half cut into wedges
- 2 tsps olive oil 1 zucchini, chopped
- 1 tsp ground cumin
- 1 tsp ground ginger
- 1/2 tsp turmeric
- 1/2 tsp ground nutmeg
- A pinch of salt
- 4 tbsps capers
- 2 tbsps chopped green olives
- 2 garlic clove, pressed
- 4 tbsps fresh mint, finely chopped
- 4 cups spinach, chopped

Procedure:

1. First, warm olive oil in a skillet over medium heat.
2. Then, place the zucchini and sauté for 10 minutes.
3. Now, stir in cumin, ginger, turmeric, nutmeg, and salt.

4. Then, pour in lemon zest, lemon juice, capers, garlic, and mint, cook for 2 minutes more.
5. Now, divide the spinach between serving plates and top with the zucchini mixture.
6. Finally, garnish with lemon wedges and olives.

Homemade Indian-Style Naan Salad

Servings: 6

Preparation Time: 10 minutes

Per Serving: Calories: 328; Fat: 17.3g; Carbs: 36.6g; Protein: 6.9g

Ingredients:

- 1 teaspoon cumin seeds
- 1 teaspoon mustard seeds
- 2 teaspoons ginger, peeled and minced
- 1 teaspoon mixed peppercorns
- 6 tablespoons sesame oil
- Himalayan salt, to taste
- 4 tomatoes, chopped
- 2 tablespoons soy sauce
- 2 tablespoons curry leaves
- 6 naan breads, broken into bite-sized pieces
- 2 shallots, chopped

Procedure:

1. First, heat 2 tablespoons of the sesame oil in a nonstick skillet over a moderately high heat.
2. Now, sauté the ginger, cumin seeds, mustard seeds, mixed peppercorns and curry leaves for 1 minute or so, until fragrant.

3. Then, stir in the naan breads and continue to cook, stirring periodically, until golden-brown and well coated with the spices.
4. After, place the shallot and tomatoes in a salad bowl; toss them with the salt, soy sauce and the remaining 2 tablespoons of the sesame oil.
5. Now, place the toasted naan on the top of your salad and serve at room temperature. Enjoy!

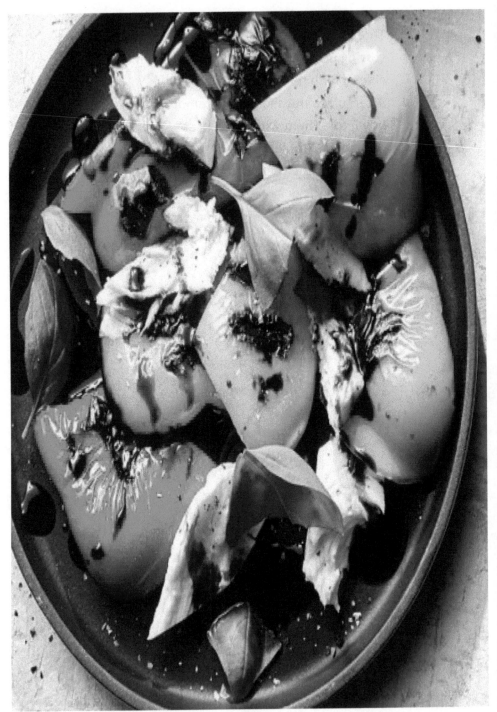

Easy Greek-Style Roasted Pepper Salad

Servings: 2

Preparation Time: 10 minutes

Per Serving: Calories: 185; Fat: 11.5g; Carbs: 20.6g; Protein: 3.7g

Ingredients:

- 4 garlic cloves, pressed
- 8 teaspoons extra-virgin olive oil
- 4 yellow bell peppers
- 2 teaspoons fresh oregano, chopped
- 2 tablespoons capers, rinsed and drained
- 4 tablespoons red wine vinegar
- 1/2 cup Kalamata olives, pitted and sliced
- 4 red bell peppers
- Seas salt and ground pepper, to taste
- 2 teaspoons fresh dill weed, chopped

Procedure:

1. First, broil the peppers on a parchment-lined baking sheet for about 10 minutes, rotating the pan halfway through the cooking time, until they are charred on all sides.
2. Then, cover the peppers with a plastic wrap to steam.
3. Discard the skin, seeds and cores.

4. Then, slice the peppers into strips and place them in a salad bowl.
5. Now, add in the remaining ingredients and toss to combine well.
6. In the end, place in your refrigerator until ready to serve. Bon appétit!

Homemade Italian Nonna's Pizza Salad

Servings: 8

Preparation Time: 15 minutes + chilling time

Per Serving: Calories: 595; Fat: 17.2g; Carbs: 93g; Protein: 16g

Ingredients:

- 2 cups marinated mushrooms, sliced
- 2 cups grape tomatoes, halved
- 2 pounds macaroni
- 1 teaspoon dried rosemary
- 8 tablespoons scallions, chopped
- 2 teaspoons garlic, minced
- 2 teaspoons dried basil
- 2 teaspoons dried oregano
- Sea salt and cayenne pepper, to taste
- 2 Italian pepper, sliced
- 1 cup black olives, sliced
- 1/2 cup extra-virgin olive oil
- 1/2 cup balsamic vinegar

Procedure:

1. First, cook the pasta according to the package directions.
2. Then, drain and rinse the pasta.
3. Let it cool completely and then, transfer it to a salad bowl.

4. Then, add in the remaining ingredients and toss until the macaroni are well coated.
5. Now, taste and adjust the seasonings; place the pizza salad in your refrigerator until ready to use. Bon appétit!

LUNCH

Homemade Roasted Apples and Cabbage

Servings: 8

Preparation Time: 15 minutes

Per Serving: Calories 127, Total Fat 7.3g, Saturated Fat 1g, Cholesterol 0mg, Sodium 4mg, Total Carbohydrate 17.8g, Dietary Fiber 3.6g, Total Sugars 12.5g, Protein 0.7g, Calcium 11mg, Iron 1mg, Potassium 170mg, Phosphorus 80mg

Ingredients:

- 4 apples - peeled, cored, and cut into 3/4-inch chunks
- Zest from 2 lemons
- 4 tablespoons olive oil, or as needed
- Juice from 2 lemons
- Salt and ground black pepper to taste
- 2 cups chopped cabbage
- pinch garlic powder to taste

Procedure:

1. First, preheat the oven to 425 degrees F.
2. Arrange cabbage in a single layer on a rimmed baking sheet; sprinkle apple pieces evenly around the baking sheet.
3. Then, drizzle the cabbage, apples with olive oil; sprinkle with salt, black pepper, and garlic powder.

4. Now, toss the mixture gently to coat.
5. Then, roast in the preheated oven until the cabbage is hot and fragrant, about 20 minutes.
6. In the end, sprinkle with lemon zest, and squeeze juice from zested lemon over the cabbage to serve.

Healthy Cabbage Bake

Servings: 8

Preparation Time: 15 minute

Per Serving: Calories 91, Total Fat 5.7g, Saturated Fat 2.5g, Cholesterol 37mg, Sodium 114mg, Total Carbohydrate 6.2g, Dietary Fiber 0.5g, Total Sugars 2.7g, Protein 3.9g, Calcium 79mg, Iron 1mg, Potassium 49mg, Phosphorus 20mg

Ingredients:

- 2 cups cabbage
- 1 cup graham crackers
- 2 cups of water
- 1 tablespoon olive oil
- 2 eggs, beaten
- 1 cup shredded Cheddar cheese

Procedure:

1. First, preheat the oven to 350 degrees F.
2. Then, bring water to boil in a medium saucepan.
3. Place chopped cabbage in the water, and return to boil.
4. Reduce heat, and simmer 2 minutes, until tender; drain.
5. Take a medium bowl, mix cabbage with oil, egg, Cheddar cheese, and 1/3 cup graham crackers.

6. Then, transfer to a medium baking dish and top with remaining graham crackers.
7. Now, cover, and bake for 25 minutes in the preheated oven, until bubbly.
8. Uncover, and continue baking 5 minutes, until lightly browned.

Homemade Zippy Zucchini

Servings: 8

Preparation Time: 10 minutes

Per Serving: Calories 80, Total Fat 5g, Saturated Fat 2.3g, Cholesterol 100mg, Sodium 159mg, Total Carbohydrate 3.7g, Dietary Fiber 1g, Total Sugars 1.9g, Protein 5.8g, Calcium 77mg, Iron 1mg, Potassium 224mg, Phosphorus 124mg

Ingredients:

- 1 medium onion
- 1/4 teaspoon salt
- 4 cups zucchini
- 1/4 teaspoon black pepper
- 4 large eggs
- 1/2 cup shredded cheddar cheese

Procedure:

1. First, cut zucchini into chunks.
2. Thinly slice the onion.
3. Now, place zucchini and onion in a 10" x 6" x 2" dish.
4. Then, cover with plastic wrap, turning one edge back slightly to vent.
5. Microwave on high for 7 minutes.
6. Drain liquid.

7. Take a large bowl, mix beaten eggs, cheese, salt, and pepper.
8. Now, add zucchini and onions, stirring well.
9. Grease dish in which vegetables were microwaved.
10. Then, pour mixture into a dish and cover with a paper towel.
11. Microwave on medium-high for 4 minutes.
12. Now, remove the paper towel and stir.
13. Continue to microwave uncovered for 4 to 6 minutes until the center is set.

Amazing Barley with Beans

Servings: 8

Preparation Time: 10 minutes

Per Serving: Calories 155, Total Fat 3.6g, Saturated Fat 0.8g, Cholesterol 2mg, Sodium 43mg, Total Carbohydrate 26.3g, Dietary Fiber 6.6g, Total Sugars 1.4g, Protein 5.8g, Calcium 43mg, Iron 2mg, Potassium 180mg, Phosphorus 120mg

Ingredients:

- 2 cups uncooked barley
- 4 cups of water
- 1/2 cup chopped onion
- 1 cup grated parmesan cheese, divided
- 2 tablespoons olive oil
- 2 cloves garlic, minced
- 4 tablespoons chopped fresh parsley
- 2 teaspoons chopped fresh basil
- 1 teaspoon black pepper
- 1 1/2 cups green beans

Procedure:

1. First, heat the oil in a saucepan over medium heat.
2. Then, stir in the barley, and cook for 2 minutes until toasted.
3. Now, pour in the water, onion, garlic, basil, and black pepper.

4. Cover, and let come to a boil.
5. Once boiling, stir in the green beans.
6. Recover, reduce heat to medium-low, and continue simmering until the barley is tender and has absorbed the water, 15 to 20 minutes.
7. After, stir in half of the parmesan cheese and the parsley until evenly mixed.
8. Now, scoop the barley into a serving dish, and sprinkle with the remaining parmesan cheese to serve.

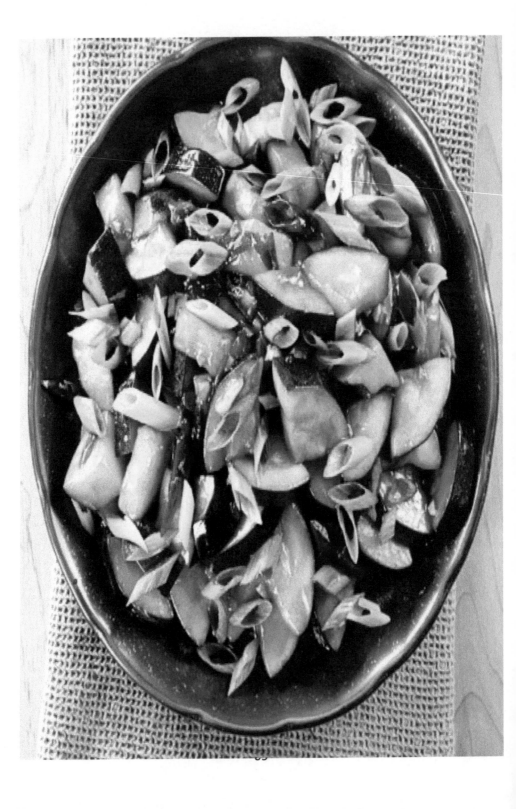

Delicious Zucchini Stir-Fry

Servings: 8

Preparation Time: 10 minutes

Per Serving: Calories 51, Total Fat 3.8g, Saturated Fat 0.6g, Cholesterol 0mg, Sodium 11mg, Total Carbohydrate 4.3g, Dietary Fiber 1.3g, Total Sugars 1.8g, Protein 1.2g, Calcium 25mg, Iron 1mg, Potassium 225mg, Phosphorus 108mg

Ingredients:

- 4 cups zucchini
- 2 tablespoons lemon juice
- 2 tablespoons olive oil
- 1/2 cup fresh parsley
- 2 teaspoons cumin
- 1 cup red onion
- 2 teaspoons black pepper

Procedure:

1. First, peel and slice zucchini and onion. Chop parsley.
2. Then, heat olive oil in a nonstick skillet over medium heat.
3. Now, sauté cumin to brown.
4. Then, add zucchini and onion and sprinkle with black pepper.
5. Stir a few times to mix.

6. After, that covers and cook for approximately 5 minutes to medium tenderness, stirring a few times.
7. Then, add lemon juice and chopped parsley.
8. Finally, mix, cook another minute, and serve.

Homemade Tofu Loaf with Nuts

Servings: 8

Preparation Time: 65 minutes

Ingredients:

- 8 garlic cloves, minced
- 2 lbs firm tofu, pressed and crumbled
- 4 tbsps olive oil + extra for brushing
- 1 cup tomato sauce
- 4 tbsps soy sauce
- 1 tsp pure date syrup
- 4 white onions, finely chopped
- 1 1/2 cups chopped mixed nuts
- 1/2 cup flaxseed meal
- 2 tbsps sesame seeds
- 2 cups chopped mixed bell peppers
- Salt and black pepper to taste
- 2 tbsps Italian seasoning

Procedure:

1. First, preheat the oven to 350 F and grease a loaf pan with olive oil.
2. Then, heat 1 tbsp of olive oil in a small skillet and sauté the onion and garlic until softened and fragrant, 2 minutes.
3. Now, pour the onion mixture into a large bowl and mix with the tofu, soy sauce, nuts, flaxseed meal,

sesame seeds, bell peppers, salt, black pepper, Italian seasoning, and date syrup until well combined.

4. Then, spoon the mixture into the loaf pan, press to fit and spread the tomato sauce on top.
5. Now, bake the tofu loaf in the oven for 45 minutes to 1 hour or until well compacted.
6. In the end, remove the loaf pan from the oven, invert the tofu loaf onto a chopping board, and cool for 5 minutes.
7. Finally, slice and serve warm.

Easy Mexican-Style Soy Chorizo & Rice Bowls

Servings: 8

Preparation Time: 50 minutes

Ingredients:

- 4 cups chopped soy chorizo
- 2 tsps taco seasoning
- 4 green bell peppers, sliced
- 2 cups brown rice
- 4 tbsps olive oil
- 2 (14 oz.) cans sweet corn kernels
- 4 cups vegetable broth
- 4 tbsps freshly chopped parsley
- 4 green onions, chopped
- 1/2 cup salsa
- 2 lemons, zested and juiced
- 2 (16 oz.) cans pinto beans, drained

Procedure:

1. First, heat the olive oil in a medium pot and cook the soy chorizo until golden brown, 5 minutes.
2. Now, season with the taco seasoning and stir in the bell peppers; cook until the peppers slightly soften, 3 minutes.
3. Then, stir in the brown rice, vegetable broth, salt, salsa, and lemon zest.

4. Close the lid and cook the food until the rice is tender and all the liquid is absorbed, 15 to 25 minutes.
5. Now, mix in the lemon juice, pinto beans, corn kernels, and green onions.
6. Allow warming for 3-5 minutes and dish the food.
7. Lastly garnish with the parsley and serve.

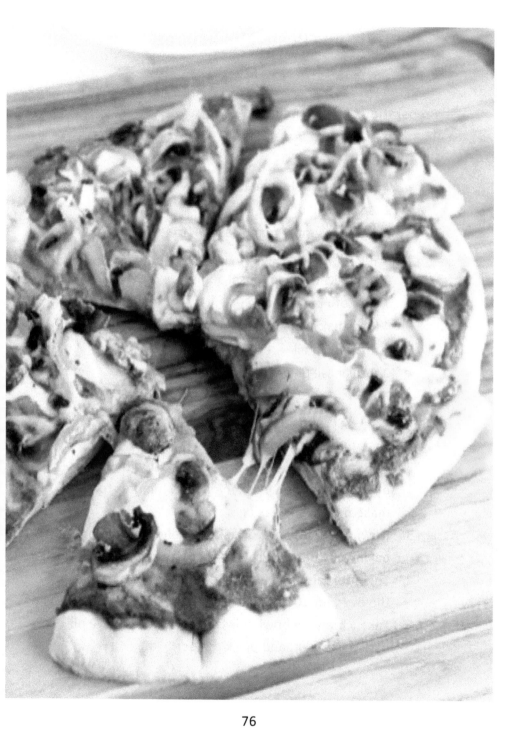

Delicious Pesto Mushroom Pizza

Servings: 8

Preparation Time: 40 minutes

Ingredients:

- 1 1/2 cups whole-wheat flour
- 2 tsps baking powder
- 1 1/2 cups grated plant-based Parmesan
- 1 cup red pizza sauce
- 2 cups sliced mixed mushrooms
- 1 cup tofu mayonnaise
- 4 tbsps flax seed powder
- 4 tbsps olive oil
- 2 tbsps basil pesto

Procedure:

1. First, preheat the oven to 350 F.
2. Take a bowl, mix the flax seed powder with 6 tbsps of water and allow thickening for 5 minutes to make the vegan "flax egg."
3. Now, mix in tofu mayonnaise, whole-wheat flour, baking powder, and salt until dough forms.
4. Then, spread the dough on a pizza pan and bake in the oven for 10 minutes or until the dough sets.
5. Take a medium bowl, mix the mushrooms, olive oil, basil pesto, salt, and black pepper.

6. Now, remove the pizza crust spread the pizza sauce on top.
7. Then, scatter mushroom mixture on the crust and top with plant-based Parmesan cheese.
8. Now, bake further until the cheese melts and the mushrooms soften, 10-15 minutes.
9. In the end, remove the pizza, slice, and serve.

Amazing Tomato & Alfredo Fettuccine

Servings: 8

Preparation Time: 20 minutes

Ingredients:

- 6 tbsps plant butter
- 2 large garlic cloves, minced
- Chopped fresh parsley to garnish
- 4 cups almond milk
- 1/2 cup halved cherry tomatoes
- 3 cups vegetable broth
- 1 1/2 cups grated plant-based Parmesan
- 32 oz. whole-wheat fettuccine
- 1 cup coconut cream

Procedure:

1. First, bring almond milk, vegetable broth, butter, and garlic to a boil in a large pot, 5 minutes.
2. Then, mix in the fettuccine and cook until tender while frequently tossing for about 10 minutes.
3. Now, mix in coconut cream, tomatoes, plant Parmesan cheese, salt, and pepper.
4. Then, cook for 3 minutes or until the cheese melts.
5. In the end, garnish with some parsley and serve warm.

Homemade Easy Braised Green Beans

Servings: 8

Preparation Time: 15 minutes

Ingredients:

- 2 carrots, cut into matchsticks
- 8 tablespoons olive oil
- 2 bay laurel
- Sea salt and ground black pepper, to taste
- 3 cups vegetable broth
- 2 lemons, cut into wedges
- 3 pounds green beans, trimmed
- 8 garlic cloves, peeled

Procedure:

1. First, heat the olive oil in a saucepan over medium flame.
2. Once hot, fry the carrots and green beans for about 5 minutes, stirring periodically to promote even cooking.
3. Then, add in the garlic and bay laurel and continue sautéing an additional 1 minute or until fragrant.
4. Now, add in the broth, salt and black pepper and continue to simmer, covered, for about 9 minutes or until the green beans are tender.
5. Taste, adjust the seasonings and serve with lemon wedges. Bon appétit!

Healthy Braised Kale with Sesame Seeds

Servings: 8

Preparation Time: 10 minutes

Per Serving: Calories: 247; Fat: 19.9g; Carbs: 13.9g; Protein: 8.3g

Ingredients:

- 2 cups vegetable broth
- 2 pounds of kale, cleaned, tough stems removed, torn into pieces
- 8 tablespoons olive oil
- 12 garlic cloves, chopped
- 2 teaspoons paprika
- Kosher salt and ground black pepper, to taste
- 8 tablespoons sesame seeds, lightly toasted

Procedure:

1. Take a saucepan, bring the vegetable broth to a boil; add in the kale leaves and turn the heat to a simmer.
2. Then, cook for about 5 minutes until kale has softened; reserve.
3. Now, heat the oil in the same saucepan over medium heat.
4. Once hot, sauté the garlic for about 30 seconds or until aromatic.

5. Then, add in the reserved kale, paprika, salt and black pepper and let it cook for a few minutes more or until heated through.
6. Finally, garnish with lightly toasted sesame seeds and serve immediately. Bon appétit!

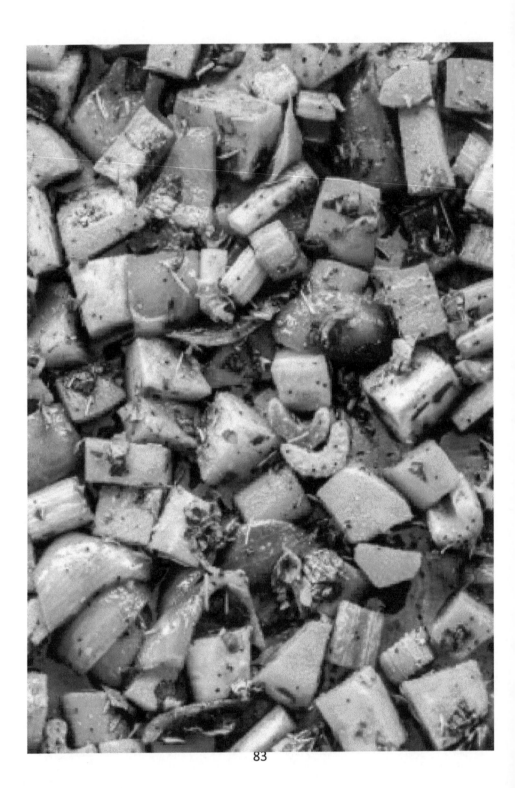

Amazing Winter Roasted Vegetables

Servings: 8

Preparation Time: 45 minutes

Per Serving: Calories: 255; Fat: 14g; Carbs: 31g; Protein: 3g

Ingredients:

- 1 pound carrot, slice into 1-inch chunks
- 1 pound parsnips, slice into 1-inch chunks
- 1 pound celery, slice into 1-inch chunks
- 1 pound sweet potatoes, slice into 1-inch chunks
- 2 large onions, slice into wedges
- 1/2 cup olive oil
- 2 teaspoons red pepper flakes
- 2 teaspoons dried basil
- 2 teaspoons dried oregano
- 2 teaspoons dried thyme
- Sea salt and freshly ground black pepper

Procedure:

1. Start by preheating your oven to 420 degrees F.
2. Then, toss the vegetables with the olive oil and spices.
3. Arrange them on a parchment-lined roasting pan.
4. Now, roast for about 25 minutes.
5. Then, stir the vegetables and continue to cook for 20 minutes more.

Delicious Traditional Moroccan Tagine

Servings: 8

Preparation Time: 30 minutes

Per Serving: Calories: 258; Fat: 12.2g; Carbs: 31g; Protein: 8.1g

Ingredients:

- 6 tablespoons olive oil
- 2 large shallots, chopped
- 2 teaspoons ginger, peeled and minced
- 8 garlic cloves, chopped
- 4 medium carrots, trimmed and chopped
- 4 medium parsnips, trimmed and chopped
- 4 medium sweet potatoes, peeled and cubed
- Sea salt and ground black pepper, to taste
- 2 teaspoons hot sauce
- 2 teaspoons fenugreek
- 1 teaspoon saffron
- 1 teaspoon caraway
- 4 large tomatoes, pureed
- 8 cups vegetable broth
- 2 lemons, cut into wedges

Procedure:

1. Take a Dutch oven, heat the olive oil over medium heat.

2. Once hot, sauté the shallots for 4 to 5 minutes, until tender.
3. Then, sauté the ginger and garlic for about 40 seconds or until aromatic.
4. Now, add in the remaining ingredients, except for the lemon and bring to a boil.
5. Immediately turn the heat to a simmer.
6. Then, let it simmer for about 25 minutes or until the vegetables have softened.
7. Lastly serve with fresh lemon

DINNER

Easy Sautéed Cauliflower with Sesame Seeds

Servings: 8

Preparation Time: 15 minutes

Per Serving: Calories: 217; Fat: 17g; Carbs: 13.2g; Protein: 7.1g

Ingredients:

- 2 cups vegetable broth
- 3 pounds cauliflower florets
- 8 tablespoons olive oil
- 4 scallion stalks, chopped
- 8 garlic cloves, minced
- Sea salt and freshly ground black pepper, to taste
- 4 tablespoons sesame seeds, lightly toasted

Procedure:

1. Take a large saucepan, bring the vegetable broth to a boil; Then,, add in the cauliflower and cook for about 6 minutes or until fork-tender; reserve.
2. Then, heat the olive oil until sizzling; Now, sauté the scallions and garlic for about 1 minute or until tender and aromatic.
3. Now, add in the reserved cauliflower, followed by salt and black pepper; continue to simmer for about 5 minutes or until heated through
4. Lastly garnish with toasted sesame seeds and serve immediately.

Homemade Mexican Quinoa Bowl

Servings: 4

Preparation Time: 25 minutes

Per Serving: Calories: 140 Cal Fat: 0.9 g Carbs: 27.1 g
Protein: 6.3 g Fiber: 6.2 g

Ingredients:

- 2 cups quinoa
- 2 cups salsa, any store brand
- 2 cups Water
- 2, 30 ounces of can black beans, thoroughly drained and rinsed
- 4 cups corn kernels, thawed if using frozen
- Sea Salt and Pepper
- 2 lime, zested and juiced
- 1 cup cilantro, chopped
- 2 romaine lettuce hearts, chopped
- 1 pint grape tomato, sliced lengthwise
- 1 cup Red Onion, diced
- 2 Avocadoes, sliced

Procedure:

1. First, add quinoa, salsa, water, beans, corn, sea salt, and pepper to the instant pot.
2. Close lid and seal.
3. Then, press the Rice button or cook on a manual setting for 12 minutes on low pressure.

4. When done cooking, allow pressure to release on its own.
5. Now, remove lid and fluff quinoa with a fork.
6. After, add lime zest and juice, cilantro, and more salt and pepper if needed.
7. Toss well.
8. Lastly serve warm and top with lettuce, tomatoes, red onion, and avocado.

Healthy Vegan Mac And Cheese

Servings: 12

Preparation Time: 13 minutes

Per Serving: Calories: 140 Cal Fat: 0.9 g Carbs: 27.1 g Protein: 6.3 g Fiber: 6.2 g

Ingredients:

- 2 pounds dry macaroni or any dry short pasta
- 8 cups water
- 3 cups unsweetened plain almond milk
- 4 tablespoons all-purpose flour or tapioca starch
- 4-6 cups shredded vegan cheese
- sea salt
- 4 tablespoons vegan butter
- 4 tablespoons mustard powder or nutritional yeast

Procedure:

1. First, add macaroni or other dry pasta, water, and salt to the instant pot.
2. Then, close lid and seal.
3. On the manual setting, set to 4 minutes.
4. While the instant pot is cooking, whisk almond milk and flour or tapioca starch until combined.
5. Set aside.
6. When done, quick release valve and open when steam is gone.
7. Then, turn instant pot on sauté mode.

8. Now, stir in almond milk and flour mixture, vegan butter, cheese, mustard powder, or nutritional yeast.
9. Stir well.
10. When the cheese is melted, turn off the instant pot, taste and add more salt if needed, serve and enjoy!

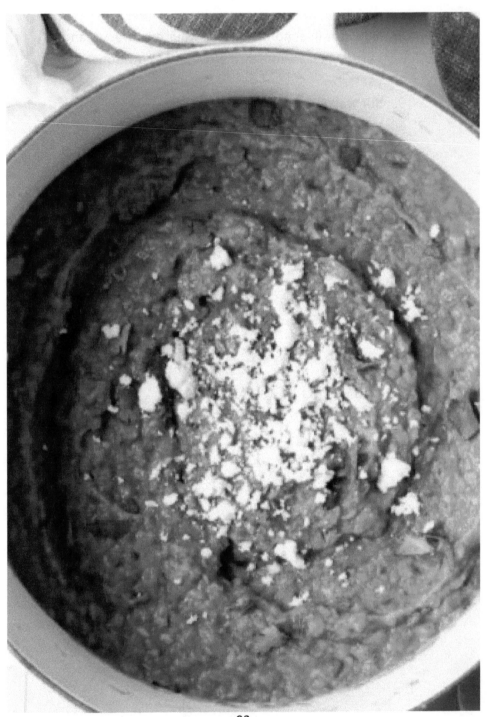

Tasty Refried Beans

Servings: 16

Preparation Time: 55 minutes

Per Serving: Calories: 140 Cal Fat: 0.9 g Carbs: 27.1 g
Protein: 6.3 g Fiber: 6.2 g

Ingredients:

- 4 tablespoons olive oil
- 4 cups onions, diced
- 12 cloves of garlic, minced
- 4 jalapenos, seeds removed and minced
- Sea salt
- Pinch cayenne pepper(optional
- 4 pounds dry black or pinto beans, thoroughly rinsed
- 24 cups vegetable broth or water
- 4 teaspoons cumin
- 4 tablespoons chili powder
- 4 teaspoons oregano
- Fresh cilantro, chopped

Procedure:

1. On the sauté setting, heat oil and add onions, garlic, jalapenos, and sea salt, and cayenne pepper (optional).
2. Now, cook for 3-4 minutes until soft and browned.

3. Then, add beans, vegetable broth or water, cumin, chili powder, and oregano to the instant pot.
4. Cover with lid and secure.
5. On the bean/chili mode, cook for 45 minutes or manual mode, high pressure for 35 minutes.
6. When done, allow the pressure to release naturally or use the quick release.
7. Now, reserve 5 cups of liquid and drain the rest.
8. Use a potato masher and mash to desired consistency. If using a blender, add beans and blend with reserved liquid.
9. Then, stir in cilantro.
10. Now, serve warm.

Homemade Cajun Vegan Shrimps

Servings: 12

Preparation Time: 10 minutes

Per Serving: Calories: 140 Cal Fat: 0.9 g Carbs: 27.1 g
Protein: 6.3 g Fiber: 6.2 g

Ingredients:

- 1 cup of coconut oil
- 1 cup chopped onion
- 1 cup chopped carrots
- 20 oz. vegan shrimps
- 2 green bell peppers, seeded, chopped
- 1/2 cup all-purpose flour
- 2 cups of water
- 8 tablespoons lemon juice
- Salt and pepper, to taste
- 6 cloves garlic
- 4 teaspoons Cajun seasoning
- 1/2 cup chopped cilantro
- 8 cups cooked brown rice, to serve with

Procedure:

1. First, heat coconut oil in an Instant pot on Sauté.
2. Now, add vegetables and cook for 5 minutes.
3. Sprinkle veggies with flour and cook for 1 minute.

4. Then, add water and stir until smooth.
5. Now, add remaining ingredients, except the rice, and season to taste.
6. Then, cover and select Manual.
7. High-pressure 4 minutes.
8. Use a quick pressure release method.
9. Finally, serve over rice.

Tasty Eggplant & Hummus Pizza

Servings: 4

Preparation Time: 25 minutes

Ingredients:

- 1 eggplant, sliced
- 1 red onion, sliced
- 2 cups cherry tomatoes, halved
- 6 tbsps chopped black olives
- Salt to taste
- Drizzle olive oil
- 4 prebaked pizza crusts
- 1 cup hummus
- 4 tbsps oregano

Procedure:

1. First, preheat oven to 390 F,
2. Take a bowl, combine the eggplant, onion, tomatoes, olives, and salt.
3. Then, toss to coat.
4. Now, sprinkle with some olive oil.
5. Arrange the crusts on a baking sheet and spread the hummus on each pizza.
6. Then, top with the eggplant mixture.
7. Bake for 20-30 minutes.
8. Finally, serve warm.

Easy Steamed Broccoli with Hazelnuts

Servings: 8

Preparation Time: 20 minutes

Ingredients:

- 2 lbs broccoli, cut into florets
- 4 tbsps olive oil
- 6 garlic cloves, minced
- 2 cups sliced white mushrooms
- 1/2 cup dry white wine
- 4 tbsps minced fresh parsley
- Salt and black pepper to taste
- 1 cup slivered toasted hazelnuts

Procedure:

1. First, steam the broccoli for 8 minutes or until tender. Remove and set aside.
2. Now, heat 1 tbsp of oil in a skillet over medium heat.
3. Then, add in garlic and mushrooms and sauté for 5 minutes until tender.
4. Now, pour in the wine and cook for 1 minute.
5. After, that stirs in broccoli, parsley, salt, and pepper.

6. Now, cook for 3 minutes, until the liquid has reduced.
7. Then, remove to a bowl and add in the remaining oil and hazelnuts and toss to coat.
8. Lastly, serve warm.

Homemade Citrus Asparagus

Servings: 8

Preparation Time: 15 minutes

Ingredients:

- 2 onions, minced
- 4 tsps lemons zest
- 2/3 cup fresh lemon juice
- 2 tbsps olive oil
- Salt and black pepper to taste
- 2 lbs asparagus, trimmed

Procedure:

1. First, combine the onion, lemon zest, lemon juice, and oil in a bowl.
2. Now, sprinkle with salt and pepper.
3. Then, let sit for 5-10 minutes.
4. Insert a steamer basket and 1 cup of water in a pot over medium heat.
5. Now, place the asparagus on the basket and steam for 4-5 minutes until tender but crispy.
6. Then, leave to cool for 10 minutes, then, arrange on a plate.
7. Finally, serve drizzled with the dressing.

Traditional Japanese-Style Tofu with Haricots Vert

Servings: 8

Preparation Time: 25 minutes

Ingredients:

- 2 cups haricots vert
- 2 tbsps grapeseed oil
- 2 onions, minced
- 10 shiitake mushroom caps, sliced
- 2 tsps grated fresh ginger
- 6 green onions, minced
- 16 oz. firm tofu, crumbled
- 4 tbsps soy sauce
- 6 cups hot cooked rice
- 2 tbsps toasted sesame oil
- 2 tbsps toasted sesame seeds

Procedure:

1. Start by placing the haricots in boiled salted water and cook for 10 minutes until tender.
2. Now, drain and set aside.
3. Then, heat the oil in a skillet over medium heat.
4. Now, place in onion and cook for 3 minutes until translucent.
5. Then, add in mushrooms, ginger, green onions, tofu, and soy sauce.

6. Now, cook for 10 minutes.
7. Share into 4 bowls and top with haricot and tofu mixture.
8. After, sprinkle with sesame oil.
9. Finally, serve garnished with sesame seeds.

Delicious Raisin & Orzo Stuffed Tomatoes

Servings: 8

Preparation Time: 40 minutes

Ingredients:

- 4 cups cooked orzo
- Salt and black pepper to taste
- 6 green onions, minced
- 2/3 cups golden raisins
- 2 tsps orange zest
- 8 large ripe tomatoes
- 2/3 cup toasted pine nuts
- ½ cup minced fresh parsley
- 4 tsps olive oil

Procedure:

1. First, preheat oven to 380 F.
2. Now, mix the orzo, green onions, raisins, and orange zest in a bowl.
3. Set aside.
4. Then, slice the top of the tomato by ½-inch and take out the pulp.
5. Now, cut the pulp and place it in a bowl.
6. After, that stirs in orzo mixture, pine nuts, parsley, salt, and pepper.

7. Now, spoon the mixture into the tomatoes and arrange on a greased baking tray.
8. Then, sprinkle with oil and cover with foil.
9. Bake for 15 minutes.
10. Uncover and bake for another 5 minutes until golden.

Homemade Rosemary Baked Potatoes with Cherry Tomatoes

Servings: 10

Preparation Time: 65 minutes

Ingredients:

- 10 russet potatoes, sliced
- 1 cup cherry tomatoes, halved
- 4 tbsps rosemary
- 4 tbsps olive oil
- Salt and black pepper to taste

Procedure:

1. First, preheat oven to 390 F.
2. Now, make several incisions with a fork in each potato.
3. Then, rub each potato and cherry tomatoes with olive oil and sprinkle with salt, rosemary, and pepper.
4. Then, arrange on a baking dish and bake for 50-60 minutes.
5. Once ready, transfer to a rack and allow to completely cool before serving.

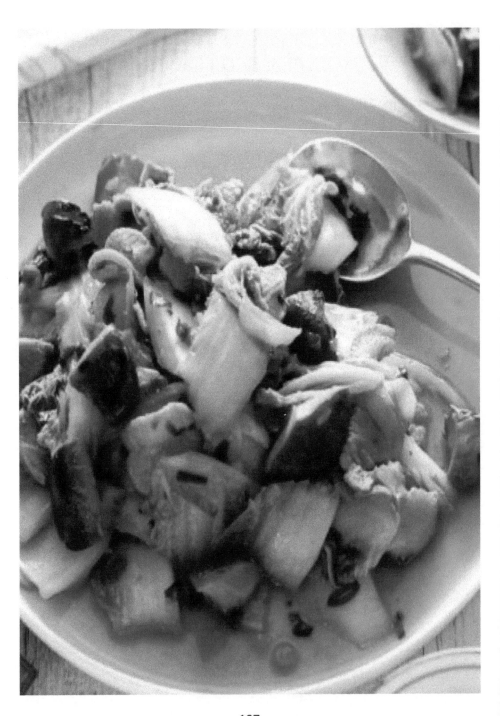

Special Chinese Cabbage Stir-Fry

Servings: 6

Preparation Time: 10 minutes

Per Serving: Calories: 228; Fat: 20.7g; Carbs: 9.2g; Protein: 4.4g

Ingredients:

- 6 tablespoons sesame oil
- 2 pounds Chinese cabbage, sliced
- 1 teaspoon Chinese five-spice powder
- Kosher salt, to taste
- 1 teaspoon Szechuan pepper
- 4 tablespoons soy sauce
- 6 tablespoons sesame seeds, lightly toasted

Procedure:

1. Take a wok, heat the sesame oil until sizzling.
2. Now, stir fry the cabbage for about 5 minutes.
3. Now, stir in the spices and soy sauce and continue to cook, stirring frequently, for about 5 minutes more, until the cabbage is crisp-tender and aromatic.
4. Finally, sprinkle sesame seeds over the top and serve immediately.